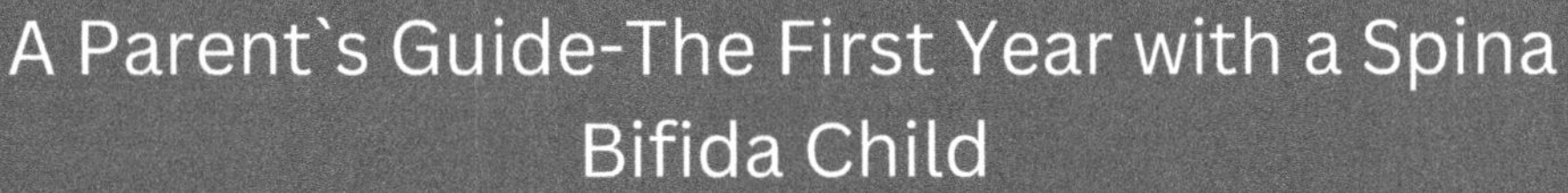

A Parent`s Guide-The First Year with a Spina Bifida Child

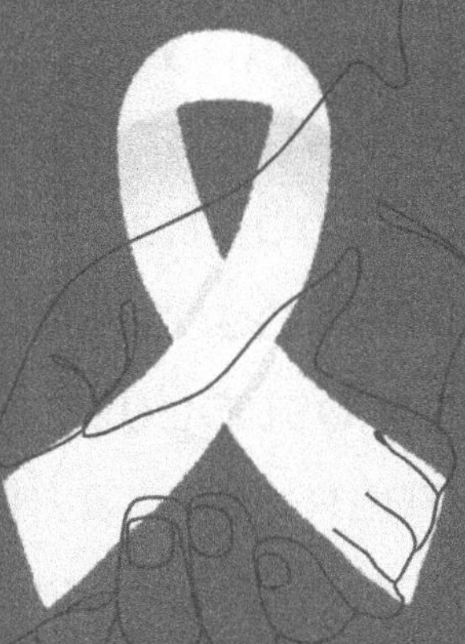

Katarina Sinor

Note to Reader

If you have picked up this book, then you are either expecting a child with spina bifida or already have a child with spina bifida and need guidance. This book has been written specifically for that purpose, as a guide, to hopefully answer most questions and get you through the first years with a little ease. This is based on my personal experience with my son who has myelomeningocele and research that I conducted for my knowledge that I want to share.

Table of Contents

Chapter 1- The Diagnosis

So here we are! You are 20-22 weeks pregnant, and you go into your anatomy ultrasound scan just a regular checkup, and find out your child has Spina Bifida. You are left wondering what it is. What does that mean for me and my child? A million questions and not enough answers or all the answers are too vague. In this chapter, I will discuss Spina Bifida and what it is. I will explain the three different types that there are and what they mean in layperson terms without all the doctor and medical jargon.

Spina Bifida is a neural tube defect that can occur anywhere along the spinal column. This means that there is a problem in the spinal column and possibly spinal cord damage as well. This problem is often caused in development when the spine is formed the neural tube does not close completely and the backbone that protects the spine doesn't form and can cause damage to the spinal cord and the nerves. The severity of the condition ranges depending on the location of the opening, the size of the opening, and the type of spina bifida. The Three most common types are Myelomeningocele, Meningocele, and Spina Bifida Occulta.

Myelomeningocele is the most serious type of spina bifida because with this condition part of the spinal cord is outside of the body and in a fluid-filled sac on the back. The fluid-filled sac is the spinal fluid that is escaping the spinal column. This causes damage to the cord and the nerves and causes moderate to severe disabilities both physical and possibly mental. Meningocele occurs when there is a fluid-filled sac, but the spinal cord is not in the sac and there is little to no damage to the spinal cord, and this can cause minor disabilities.

Lastly, there is the Spina Bifida Occulta. This type of Spina Bifida is the least severe and is described as hidden because it is not often seen or diagnosed. It occurs when there is a small gap in the spine, but no major opening and no sac on the back. The spinal cord nerves are usually normal and do not cause many disabilities if any. Usually, just a tuft of hair can be found at the site of the spina bifida occulta.

Now that you know the different types of spina bifida that can occur, let's talk about what it all means.

Chapter 2- Spina bifida- What does it mean?

You received the diagnosis that your child has spina bifida, you know what it is now, but what does it mean for you and your child`s future? It simply means that there may or may not need to be adjustments. Adjustments to the rest of your pregnancy, delivery, postpartum, your child`s life, and possibly your original plan or what you had in mind for what your new life was going to look like.

Since you have received your diagnosis, you will now be a high-risk pregnancy. This means that you will be monitored frequently with ultrasounds, heart rate monitors, and more frequent Obstetrics follow-ups. There is a Blood test that can be performed to confirm the spina bifida and that is called an AFP. This test is used to measure proteins that are produced by the baby that are passed to the mother's bloodstream. This blood test is also not 100% accurate but can aid in the diagnosis confirmation. This helps to further look at and determine the neural tube defect and other issues.

There is the option to also check the amniotic fluid by removing some of the fluid in a procedure called amniocentesis to help with the confirmation of the diagnosis. Since you are a high-risk pregnancy, you will also need to deliver at the hospital and may need to deliver via c-section depending on the severity of the child`s condition and the physical state of the mother. The child will also in turn spend some time in the Neonatal Intensive Care Unit and may need to have surgeries early in life.

Chapter 3- Pregnancy, Delivery, Postpartum

Pregnancy, Delivery, and Postpartum are all going to look different than what you may have originally planned or wanted. Your pregnancy will consist of more doctors' appointments, blood tests, ultrasounds, and scans than a low-risk pregnancy. This does not mean that you cannot enjoy your pregnancy it simply means a little more time spent taking care of the medical necessities. Some mothers and babies qualify for a procedure called in-utero fetal surgery, in which the mom has a c-section and just the child`s area of the defect is exposed to be repaired.

The defect is repaired, and the baby and mom are left to heal and recover, this surgery can allow a higher chance of less nerve damage or fewer difficulties for the child. However, after this surgery is conducted, Mom does have to rest effectively and is on bed rest for some time to recover. As with any surgery, this is not 100% successful and is up to each individual and their medical care team as to what decision is made regarding this option.

Delivery is something that depends on the type of spina bifida your child has as well as, what you want your body to go through. If your child has spina bifida occulta or meningocele, you may be able to deliver your child safely vaginally. However, if your child is diagnosed with Myelomeningocele, like my son, then the safest route you may find is to deliver via c-section. Now, I understand this may not be an easy decision and it certainly was not for me because I had one child delivered successfully naturally and that is what I intended this time, but it was not possible if I wanted him here safe. So, I decided to go with the Doctor`s recommendations to have him delivered via c-section and he was delivered safely.

After Delivery of the baby whether vaginally or via c-section your child may be taken to the NICU (neonatal intensive care unit) immediately after delivery. The reason for this is that the child needs to be examined quickly to determine if any immediate action or care is needed. You will then be sent to postpartum for recovery. If you had your child in the labor room you may be at the hospital for 1-2 days, but if you had your child via c-section you may be there for 4 or more days depending on insurance and if there are any complications with your recovery.

Postpartum for you may be challenging as your child will be separated from you for a while depending on the severity of the condition. From my personal experience, my son was in the NICU for almost a month, and this was very hard on me. During your postpartum period, you may be making a lot of frequent trips to the hospital to see your child due to this separation. You may also not be able to breastfeed due to the location and severity of the opening, or simply because you don't get the bonding that your body needs to develop and produce the milk. Do not be disheartened by this because the hospitals often have donor breastmilk that is specifically used to help the NICU babies and give them the nutrients they need.

Chapter 4 — First year of life

As with any child, the first year of life can be a wild and amazing adventure, but with a child that has spina bifida depending on the case, it may be even more wild. This chapter is about what you might expect in the first year and is based solely on my own experience with my spina bifida son and the research that I have conducted.

The first month is delivery, your postpartum recovery, and monitoring and recovery of your child after birth in the NICU. There are many specialists that you may encounter during this time. The specialists are there to discuss results and the status of the child`s condition as well as what is expected, answer any questions you may have, and help with scheduling appointments for future observations when discharged from the hospital.

These specialists could be Neurosurgery and Neurology because the surgery that may be conducted to repair the opening involves the nervous system. This surgery would be a spinal closure surgery in which they drain the fluid sac, place the spinal cord back in the spinal column, and then repair and close the muscular and skin area surrounding the opening. After this surgery, your child will be sent back to the NICU for continued recovery and monitoring to make sure that the closure was successful, and that the child is not building spinal fluid in the brain. If this does occur, then the child would need to have a shunt placed. This shunt is a plastic tube that runs from the brain into the abdominal cavity to redirect the excess fluid. After this surgery, the child will again be sent back to the NICU for continued monitoring and recovery.

Gastroenterology and nutrition may be another specialist that you see for monitoring gastric issues aka stomach and nutrient absorption issues. Your child may also need to see a continence clinic physician because the Spinal fluid being redirected into the abdominal cavity can cause the child to have increased acidity in the bowels, which may be painful. This increased acidity may also cause tissue breakdown around the anal area. In this scenario, you may then have to seek assistance from wound care to gain supplies and tools to care for the child's butt area more than just your traditional butt cream.

Urology and continence specialists will be used to monitor bladder, kidney, and bowel functions to avoid and aid in any complications that may arise. An Orthopedic specialist will be seen if the child needs any corrective or assistive equipment like leg braces, custom-fitted shoes, walkers, or any issues related to bone function, growth, and development. Above is just a list of the few specialists you may encounter depending on the situation you may have. These specialists will attempt to work as a team in aiding you and your child and providing the needed care for the best quality of life.

After recovery from delivery and you and your child are discharged, which may or may not be at the same time depending on severity, you then will have your usual pediatric appointments that you would for any child for their vaccinations and regular health monitoring. Though you may use the pediatric visit for illnesses and vaccinations, they may not be the person that you seek out if there are complications related to certain specialties. This is because of the child`s condition and the pediatricians not having in-depth knowledge of the condition they may refer you to reach out to your specialists if it is not a common issue related to the child`s growth and development.

The first year will also be used to establish if the child needs any assistance with daily activities and would need therapy. These therapies could be physical therapy for mobility and daily body function, occupational therapy for fine motor skills such as grabbing and picking objects up, speech therapy and feeding therapy for any oral difficulties such as swallowing or talking, and many more such as music therapy or water therapy. These therapies are used to help the child grow, develop, and improve their life skills and improve their day-to-day activities. The frequency that you attend these therapies will depend on the therapist's recommendation after evaluation and following development milestones for where the child is, where they should be, and how to get there or as close to the development milestone as possible.

This is by no means an in-depth description of all the personnel that may assist you along your journey, but it will help you to know what to expect the good, the bad, and the ugly, and who you could be working with for your child's health and happiness as well as your own mental clarity and knowledge of what to expect. Just to give a little comfort in this stage of life as well there are associations that help aid parents in their struggles and if they have questions for Spina Bifida. I will also let you know that even though I have personally faced these struggles with my child, he smiles every day and continues to give me the strength to help him in any way I can knowing that he is getting the best quality life I can offer him.

REFERENCES

1. Mayo Clinic. In Utero Spina Bifida Surgery. 1998- 2024. Mayo Foundation for Medical Education and Research. https://www.mayoclinic.org/in-utero-spina-bifida-surgery/vid-20388952

2. Centers for disease control and prevention. Spina Bifida. October 4, 2023. U.S. Department of Health and Human Services.

https://www.cdc.gov/ncbddd/spinabifida/facts.html

3. Spina Bifida Association. 2024. Spina Bifida Association of America. https://www.spinabifidaassociation.org/

4. Nemours Children`s Health. Spina Bifida. 2024. The Nemours Foundation. https://www.nemours.org/onsitesearch.html?q=spina+bifida

5. Spina Bifida of Jacksonville. 2024. Spina bifida of Jacksonville, Florida Support group. https://www.spinabifidajax.org/